I0413621

True

Stories

For

The

Physically

Challenged

Everybody is Able

Senior Partner

&

Anyaehie George

Senior Partner and George Anyaehie

ISBN: 1495982831
ISBN-13: 9781495982835

Dedication

To Doris Ngozi, a gallant soldier fighting against the enemy called disability.

Content

Acknowledgments

We are not achievers but mere receivers.

We are not great men but helped men.

We are not wise men but inspired men.

We are not strong men but strengthened men.

What I am privileged to hear is what I write.

Without my Senior Partner, I am nothing.

Anyaehie George

<u>Senior Partner and George Anyaehie</u>

Introduction

Anyaehie George

Speech Impediment

G or! gor! gor! gor! gor! gor! gor! gor! gor! gor! gor! gor And the whole students in the class echoed: "George the machine gun." I stopped talking, raised my head and looked at my class mates; almost everyone was laughing while others were mimicking me. Even our class teacher was intelligently mocking me, because he covered his face with his lesson note book, I was sure he was laughing behind it. In shame, I lowered my head, closed my eyes and cried like a baby.

What was my crime? I was only trying to answer a question thrown to the class. I had vowed never to answer or ask any question in class, but I was tempted to answer this question because our Government teacher promised to give a bonus continuous assessment score to any student who answers the question rightly. The question was: define democracy.

After a thorough fight with my thoughts, one said; "do not answer, you will be insulted" and another whispered "George you know the answer, speak." I decided to answer the question. I rigorously rehearsed what to say silently; "government of the people, by the people and for the people" and finally raised my hands. Mr. Phil pointed at me and said; "George let's hear from you." As soon as I tried to speak, I felt the normal trip over my tongue and what I could only utter was; Gor! gor! gor! gor! gor! gor! gor! gor! gor! gor! gor! gor!, until the mockery and laughter of the class halted me.

I have been a stutterer since I was born. My condition was so severe that I was compared with the dumb. I wouldn't speak until I stamp my feet on the ground, slap my laps with my hands or hit the person I was speaking to. My parents did all they could to help me. They sought diverse professional advice which they apply on me; all were ineffective. I became partially dumb because I wouldn't speak anywhere except in the mist of my close family members. My classmates nicknamed me "machine gun," because of the sound I made when I stumble. I would never ask my teachers any question, even when I needed clarifications.

However, I grew up to become a good writer. What I couldn't do with my mouth, I did with my hands. My writing was so outstanding that my teachers had to invite me to defend what I wrote because I hardly speak in the classroom. Before graduating from higher institution, I started writing and circulating motivational articles. My readers were so impressed that they invited me to speak on my writings. I wanted to attend but was afraid because I might be embarrassed. Another challenge was that most of our final year tests and examination would be oral and not written. When I discovered that I could no longer hide from the public, I decided to step out boldly.

My decision was to keep speaking anywhere regardless of the repetition, the sound or who is mocking. I started asking and answering questions in the class. Majority of my teachers became aware of my challenge, and they gave me enough time to ask and answer questions. My classmates laughed and laughed until they got tired of mocking. Most of them started listening patiently to me because I was always making sense. In no time, the class became used to me. I also discovered that my confidence level improved, and the rate of my repetition kept reducing as I kept speaking. If boldness and confidence are the cure for my disabilities, then I need to take the full dose of them, I thought. Immediately, I organized a programme for myself.

I decided that every morning, before lectures begin, I would go into any available class and speak to the students on academic success. It was a fearful decision, nevertheless; I started. The more class I spoke to, the higher my boldness and confidence and the lesser I stammered. Students began to love my speech, and soon I became well known. My final year project-defense presentation was the best, and I earned an "A."

After graduation, I packaged the academic success articles into a book. The book was successful, and I kept receiving countless invitation to speak in schools, churches and other public places. Currently, I have spoken to more than 30,000 students, and I am still speaking. Today I however stammer slightly, but I'm the best speaker anytime, anywhere and majority of my income comes from speaking.

Introductory lesson

Sometimes the best in a man is born in his effort to tackle his disabilities. Most times our uncommon qualities are hidden in our challenges. Some people esteem the magnitude of their challenges than the size of their opportunities. They allow their challenges to becloud the tangible opportunities packaged in their disabilities. Your ability to see the riches and fame wrapped in your challenges is what generates the stamina to overcome them. If you must get the honey, you must face the bees. If you say you are incapacitated, you are correct, if you say you are not, you are also right.

The truth is that; nobody is a disable. A part of your body might be disabled but you are not. The only completely disable person I know is a dead man. A disabled person is unproductive because he cannot do anything. You are only physically challenged because a part of your body is malfunctioning. A man's ability is not measured by the completeness of the parts of his body, but by the soundness of his mind. There are physical complete men who are disabled, because their minds are unproductive. A man is not incapacitated when he loses an arm, but he becomes that when he loses his mind or life. The real measure of a man's capacity is in intellectual scaling which connotes mind usage.

Those who have physical conditions that affect their ability were once referred as crippled, disabled, handicapped and crippled, all words focusing on what they could not do rather than what they can do. With practice, determination and hard work, anyone can be successful. Only the producer knows everything about his product. Anyone can say anything about the product but only the producer knows the capacity and worth of his invention. The product cannot know its capacity until it faces challenges. Without life's difficulties, you might underestimate your worth when   People can call you anything they think or feel, but they cannot change your worth. Only you and your Creator know your worth.

Therefore, if you decide to believe that you are a disable that's your business. It is better to face the difficulties of your condition, than to succumb to the threats and discrimination of bullies and the unlearned. If you refuse to face that challenge, it will remain forever. The challenge might look very mighty, but it is empty inside. All you need to do is to break in and walkover.

Relevance

Bible Naaman

Leprous

In the year 885 B.C., the people of Syria were surprise that Naaman was still the commander of the Armed forces of Syria. He was diagnosed of leprosy a highly infectious disease that can result in tissue loss causing fingers and toes to become shortened and deformed, as cartilage is absorbed into the body. At that time, there was no known cure for the disease in Syria.

In Europe during the Middle Ages, leprosy sufferers had to wear special clothing, ring bells to warn others that they were close, and even walk on a particular side of the road, depending on the direction of the wind. While in Asia, sufferers were often confined against their will in leper colonies or outside the city walls. Leprous mothers were not allowed to get close, touch or breastfeed their babies out of fear that they could infect them.

The people of Syria expected the king to dismiss Naaman and appoint a new commander to avoid the spread of the disease in the palace and the entire city. After all, the Syrian army can boast of hundreds of valiant soldiers qualified to take Naaman's job.

However, Naaman was still dinning with the king on the same table, dishing food from the same bowl. Some of the royal physicians earlier called the attention of the king to the implication of his closeness to Naaman. The most annoying one was that the King allowed Naaman to enter the Temple of their powerful and holy gods Rimmon. And the King always bowed to their gods leaning on the leprous arm of Naaman. The people were furious, but they remained calm because he was their king.

Nevertheless, the members of the armed forces of

Syria knew why the King can never dismiss Naaman. He was an exceptional valiant soldier; through him, Syria won many battles. He kept undergoing diverse military trainings that his physical disability had no effect on his skillfulness in the battle field. The king knew that he was relevant in the kingdom. What Naaman could do, hundred gallant soldiers put together might not achieve it. In fact, he was the best soldier in the entire Syria. Therefore, the king preferred to be infected with leprosy than to lose his kingdom in the battlefields. Ostracizing Naaman was like obtaining a licence of doom for Syria.

Regardless of what some people in the kingdom said, Naaman remained relevant in Syria until he was healed of leprosy by Prophet Elisha. Resulting from the exploits of Naaman, leprous people were no longer seen as third class citizens in Syria. They were accepted and allowed to dwell within the city walls.

Lesson 1

Anything can be relevant, if only it can solve a problem or satisfy a need. A dog that solves an international problem will become a global celebrity. If a monkey discovers the cure to HIV/AIDS, that monkey will have human bodyguards. Regardless of how you are or look, just be relevant and nations will beg for your service. If you have what they want, they will beg to have it.

Find a discipline, acquire relevant training or education and be a master or an authority in that discipline, automatically, people will start sorting for your goods or services. Nobody wants to know if you are physically challenged or not, all they desire is for you to satisfy their needs. People care little of what they say about you, as long as you give the right result, people will adore you. The walls of segregation and discrimination crumble at the feet of relevance. Countries deport only irrelevant people. If you are a solution to the nation's problems, Immigration policies would be breached just to ensure that you remain in that country.

People celebrate positive impact and not appearance. The world needs medication, if you can heal her, she would give you wealth and fame regardless of your looks. Fame and wealth are not selective; they go to anyone who has the solution to problems.

Purpose

Cobhams Asuquo

Blind

I was born on the 6th of January 1981, the last of six children. My mother said that I was like other children. She said I seem perfectly normal until about three months after when she began noticing my clumsiness. My father was not always around because he was a military officer in the Nigerian Army. It was my mother who served the family in all parental capacities. She became very worried about my discomfort and decided to seek medical attention. She quickly took me to the University Teaching Hospital in Ibadan from where we were referred to a hospital in Kano. There, her worst fears were confirmed; her son had been blind in the womb, and nothing could be done to restore his sight.

From the day my mother discovered I was blind; I was never treated like a dependent. I was shown where everything I needed in the house was few times, and I was allowed to get them myself in subsequent times. Although everyone at home showered me with love and affection, they were there to answer my questions, took particular interest, but they spanked me when they thought it necessary. Childhood was interesting, and it was fun. I did everything I was big enough to do. I ran around, played with motor-tyres, jumped staircases and did all kinds of stuffs. I was just that kid who was around. I got into fights and was competitive. I was a very adventurous kid with an event filled childhood.

At age six and seven, I used to puff my cheeks and play the twelve buff blues. I also used to drum and make music with everything in the house, from the dining table to barrels of water, my chest, stomach and anything I could lay my hands on, so my mother encouraged me by buying musical toys for me. Soon people in our barracks started enjoying my beats, and I organise concerts in our neighbourhood, drumming on my mother's barrels of water.

My father played a lot of music around. When I replicated some of the songs I've heard; drumming and trying to sing them, it'll be my own style, and my audience enjoyed them. All the kids from the neighbouring block would come, and we'd hang out, and we'd make so much noise. My music talent became more evident as I grew older. I started to play the piano at about age 8 or 9. When I was nine years old, I was already playing for my church.

In their bid to make me independent, my parents sent me to boarding schools; Pacelli School for the Blind and King's College Lagos respectively. Academically, I was doing very well, and I always had good results. As a student, I regularly strolled out of school and go in and out of the studio to work on commercials, jingles and other kinds of stuff just for fun. I started meeting some of the big names in the Nigerian music industry like Faze and the Plantatun Boiz, Maintain and others. Some of them took a chance with me and liked my productions. At age 16, I started producing for some of these artistes.

My musical journey, however, seemed to come to a halt a few years later when I entered the university to pursue studies in law. I like Law, and I am fascinated by its academics and practice. I was studying Law, but I spent more time in the Music Department. I was always playing the piano and hanging out with Musicians. I was a friend with people like Darey, who was studying Music in the University of Lagos. We would hang out and play music and just have a good time. My room then was almost like a mini studio.

After three years in the University, I started sensing

that law is not my purpose. Music had always been in me, and I think it was time for me to face facts and ask myself if I was ready to be doing litigation in wig and gown or not. Soon I realized that I have to follow my musical passion, I left university to embark on a path that, for a young blind musician in Nigeria, was far from easy to tread. I had an interesting academic record. So when I opted for music, my parents knew it was out of passion and not because I was failing as far as academics were concerned.

At the beginning, it was not easy. I had to sleep on studio floors all across Lagos, worked at different studios, worked without pay. I had to convince people that I could do it. I had sessions that were cancelled because they weren't sure I could deliver either because they thought I was too young or maybe as a blind person. However, it didn't take long for me to prove myself as my musical talent soon began to shine. Over the next few years, I went on to work closely with internationally-renowned artists such as pop sensation Asa and R&B star Darey and the demand for my skill, musically, kept building. I have also produced work for Yinka Davis, the Rooftop MCs, Charlie Boy, Mode 9, Sasha, Omawunmi, Timi Dakolo, Banky W, Sound Sultan, MI, Style Plus Tuface, Timaya, and that's only about a quarter of the list. I wrote and produced work for a number of organisations as well: MTN, Zain, Globacom, Etisalat, Stanbic IBTC, Coca Cola, Close-up, Reltel and so many others. A major breakthrough came in 2005; I signed on with Sony ATV London as a songwriter and in 2008, I clinched the Hip Hop World Award Best Producer of the year.

Currently, I am raising young outstanding artistes through Cobhams Asuquo Music Production (CAMP). Some of our labelled artistes are Omolara, Bez, Joan, Pheel and Shamel. Bez's debut album 'Super Sun' was highlighted on The Boston Globe's top ten list of best 'world music' albums of 2011. I am also married, with a son.

Lesson 2

Physical disability is not purpose disability. Your bodily challenge doesn't change your purpose or passion. Your challenge is not a passport to change your passion. It shouldn't make you do anything because you are capable of doing them. You have a purpose to pursue and achieve; your physical challenge cannot change it. You must fulfill destiny regardless of the challenge you face. Physical challenge is not a permission to be pushed around by relatives and friends to do any job.

Furthermore, you don't choose a field because somebody that has the same challenge with you is in that field. Your friend is a doctor, and he is an amputee like you is not a guarantee that you will be prosperous in the medical field. You are not called to be a blind musician because Cobhams is successful. Any physically challenged person can spur you to pursue your passion and not to duplicate his own career except you are passionate about the field.

Nobody should force you to do what you don't have passion for. Allow people to encourage you to pursue your passion. You are created to do what you are designed and empowered to do and not what is available. You are created to do what you are created and empowered to do and not what your body permits you to do. Not having arms cannot disqualify you from becoming a writer. You can skilfully write with other parts of the body. Nobody should choose a career for you, follow your passion. It is your passion that fires up your vigour to pursue your purpose. You cannot succeed in every profession, except you are passionate about it.

It is passion that makes you outstanding in a field. It is never too late to start pursuing your passion. Excellent results come speedily and cheaply when you are passionate about what you do. Your stardom is tied to the actualisation of your purpose. Your fame and wealth are in your purpose no matter how simple or irrelevant it seems. It is never too late to be right.

The ability to overcome opposition as you pursue your purpose is packaged in the process of achieving just your vision. Your helpers in destiny and those that matter to your advancement are all positioned only in your area of passion. Working outside your purpose brings struggles and fruitless efforts. You'll find contentment when your talent is fully developed and your passion is wholly pursued.

Practice

Mordecai "Three Finger" Peter Brown

Amputee

Mordecai Centennial Peter Brown was born on October 19, 1876, during harvest season, in the rural mining community of Nyesville, Indiana. He was called Centennial to mark the hundredth birthday of the United States of America. Peter was his father's name, and there was an uncle named Mordecai. Mordecai had seven brothers and sisters.

In the summer of his fifth year, Mordecai and his elder brother were performing their daily chores, helping out on the farm. The boys' uncle kept livestock, and they always assisted with the feeding and care of the animals. While helping his brother to operate a feed chopper, Mordecai put his right hand under the moving blades of machinery. The feed cutter used series of circular blades that chopped the feed into pieces so that it would be easier for the animals to digest. The razor-sharp blades closed down on the fingers of his right hand, and every of his fingers were chopped to ribbons.

Dr Gillum, an experienced wartime surgeon was the town physician. He amputated the damaged finger. Several other fingers were broken and cut so he managed to sow them together, then applied splints to each finger to hold them straight while they healed. The doctor did a good job, and the injury was healing quickly.

Few weeks later with his hands wrapped in bandages, Mordecai and his sister were playing with a pet rabbit. He was making the rabbit swim in a tub partly filled with water. Suddenly, he lost balance and tumbled into the tub; his injured right hand smashed again at the bottom of the tub, breaking six bones. Afraid that his father would spank him hard, Mordecai told his sister not to tell anybody about the incident. They rebandaged Mordecai's hand and kept it secret.

Few weeks later, Dr. Gillum came to inspect his patient. When he removed the bandaged, Mordecai could no longer straighten his little finger, and the other fingers were bent and deformed. His middle finger bent first to the right and then to the left. Dr. Gillum, considered rebreaking the misaligned fingers to set them straight again, but he dismissed the notion, probably figuring that the lad had already undergone enough trauma. He decided to leave Mordecai with a permanently damaged hand.

Baseball was important in the community. There were no film theatres or many other things to do for entertainment. So after work and on weekends nearly the whole town went to the ballpark to play or watch baseball. Mordecai fell in love with the game of baseball and dreamt of becoming a baseball star. However, his disability would be difficult to overcome in the field of play. If he wants to be a hitter, it would be demanding for him to hold a bat with his damaged hand. To be a good fielder, he must be able to throw the ball without a sinking action which was not easy.

Mordecai decided to practice. He spent hours hurling rocks at the side of outbuildings attempting to knock out knotholes to improve his accuracy. He would stand at a distance from his mother's smoke house, at the point substituting a ball for a rock, and through with such force that the sphere would fly back to him. He practiced with potato; any round weighed object as same as a baseball. Hours of toss after toss, with each thump against the wooden plank of the barn, his aim got better and better. A former minor leaguer named Legs O'Connell Brown saw his determination and lectured Mordecai on baseball gripping and tossing with his injured hand.

With O'Connell's help Brown overcame the pain of handling the ball, yet time and again when he tossed it, the ball curved and jumped stubbornly, landing with an awkward twist. Brown was frustrated by this inability to control the ball, until O'Connell convinced him to turn the odd throwing style into an advantage.

With practice and perseverance, Brown learnt to pitch a natural curve ball with a special flair made possible only by the mass of crippled fingers on his right hand. Further, the way he was forced to hold the ball when he threw made it spin in a radical manner, and the extra topspin made it difficult for a batter to connect with his pitches. His pitches didn't only curve; it curved and dropped at the same time; it became extremely hard for batters to hit, and if they did hit it, they hit it into the ground because they couldn't get under it. It was as if God had moulded the perfect instrument to throw the curveball. While the two clawed fingers cradled the ball securely, he could tuck the fleshy nub of the remainder of his index finger firmly behind the baseball, giving it an unusual spin. After a few years, Mordecai became one of the best players in Nyesville and the entire baseball world. He became the mainstay of his club.

Brown finished his major-league career wining 239 and losing 130 games, with 1375 strikeouts, 2.06 Earned Run Average and 55 Shutouts, the third-best ERA in Major League Baseball. Brown was elected to baseball's Hall of Fame in 1949. In 1999, he was named as a finalist to the Major Baseball All-Century Team. And the machine that cut his fingers is displayed in Nyesville as a tourist attraction. No Cubs pitcher or team has topped his career statistics marks achievements in 100 years.

Lesson 3

One of the greatest qualities of man is adaptability. Man can function comfortably in any condition. Most times we think that an organ cannot replace another, but the truth is that most part of our bodies can comfortably perform the functions of another. The legs can serve as the arms. We can move with some parts of our body apart from the legs. Our smell can see, and our eyes can speak. The ineffectiveness of an organ ignites the genius in another. Nature ensures that everyone extract equally from her resources. If an individual is deaf nature ensures that his eyes, mouth, feel, or any part of his body becomes extraordinary to ensure fairness. Therefore, nobody is disadvantaged because life is just.

It is also important to note that it is not the effectiveness of all the organs of the body that guarantees success or greatness but the rare features of an organ. Great Singers have uncommon voices, and celebrated soccer stars possess exceptional legs.

However, many have failed to discover and tap the riches of their extraordinary qualities because of the pains of practice. The only price for mastery is practice. The agony of practice is the fuel of professionalism. The gain of mastery is far greater than the pains of practice. It might be painful but it will soon be gainful. Training is normally painful at the initial stage; if you persevere, the pains will reduce gradually and later disappear.

Enduring the pains of practice is the only channel of overcoming the menace called; disability. Practice is the sole means of tapping the hidden extraordinary abilities in you. With diligent practice, you can do what you think you can't.

Comfort Zone

Franklin D. Roosevelt

Polio

In the summer of 1921, Franklin D. Roosevelt and his family took a holiday to their summer home on Campobello Island, off the coast of Maine and New Brunswick. Frank needed this vacation badly, after a very hectic political adventure. In 1920, he received nomination from his party, the Democrats to run as the vice presidential candidate with, Governor James M. Cox of Ohio as the presidential candidate. Although, the Cox-Roosevelt ticket was defeated by Republican Warren G. Harding in the presidential election by a wide margin, but it was a good political point for Franklin.

On August 10, 1921, after a day spent outdoors,

Roosevelt began to feel weak. He went to bed early but woke up the next day much worse, with a high fever; his temperature hovered at 102 degrees and with pain in his lower back and legs. By August 12, 1921, he could no longer stand. His wife; Eleanor called a number of doctors to come and see FDR, but it wasn't until August 25 that Dr. Robert Lovett diagnosed him with poliomyelitis. At age 39, Roosevelt lost the use of both of his legs. It was a terrible blow to the Roosevelt family. Everybody knew that it was the end of the political career of Franklin.

Sara Roosevelt, Franklin's mother has been Franklin's driving force all through his life. Franklin always obeyed her commands. She was rich and very influential. Sara instructed her only son to retire from politics and return to the family estate at Hyde Park to live as a gentleman invalid. Sara Roosevelt, like most people at the time, believed that disabled persons had no place in public, and that the most appropriate future for her son was to retire quietly to Hyde Park.

Truly, Franklin would be very comfortable in the family estate; he would be well taken care of. His rich mother could support him financially and in other aspects. He would also inherit a large estate after his mother's death. Hyde Park was the safest and most comfortable place to stay for Franklin. Venturing into politics on a wheelchair would be suicidal because opposition will capitalize on his physical challenge. If able-bodied men failed in politics what would be the fate of Franklin? After all Franklin has scored some remarkable political points. He has served as a senator for two terms and was appointed by President Woodrow Wilson as the Assistant Secretary of the Navy. He has also been a Vice Presidential candidate. He could just retire from politics; continue his legal profession, business and hobby of stamp collection. This was the most convenient decision for him.

However, Franklin Roosevelt abandoned his mother's proposed comfort zone. For seven years, Franklin stayed out of active politics. He was busy preparing himself for his re-emergence in the political world of the United States of America. Roosevelt refused to be limited by his impairment.

To overcome his lack of mobility, Roosevelt acquired steel and later duraluminun leg braces that could be locked into an upright position to keep his legs straight. With the 7lbs. apiece leg braces on under his clothes, Roosevelt could stand and slowly walk with the aid of clutches and a companion's arm. Roosevelt even had his car adapted to his disability by installing hand controls rather than foot pedals so that he could sit behind the wheel and drive. He also maintained his political contacts largely through correspondence and through the increasing public activities of his wife. He also mended fences with the Democratic Party. He even assisted Alfred E. Smith win the election for governor of New York in 1922. He also made friends in the press.

Despite his pains, he kept his humour and charisma. In 1928, when he nominated Smith for president, he dragged himself laboriously to the podium without crutches, one hand holding a cane and the other clutching his son's arm to give a speech. It was an important personal triumph, signaling his readiness to resume an active political career; Roosevelt knew that for him to come back to politics successful, he needed to convince the public that he was getting better. And that was exactly what he did.

Sure of his political packaging and marketability, Franklin Roosevelt re-entered politics in 1928 as a Governorship aspirant of the Democratic Party. Roosevelt won the election in 1928 for governor of New York and then won again in 1930. Roosevelt's strong base in the most populous state made him an obvious candidate for the Democratic presidential nomination. In the election of 1932, citizens were demanding change and Franklin promised it to them. In a landslide election, Franklin D. Roosevelt won the presidency. Before Franklin became president, there was no limit to the number of terms a person could serve as president of the United States. He served for 12 years (four terms) until his death in 1945, the only president ever to do so, and a central figure in world events during the mid-20th century, leading the United States during a time of worldwide economic depression and total war.

Lesson 4

It was 8am, in a typical African community. Everything was stepping out of their resting place to seek for the day's bread. Humans are seen riding or walking to their place of work. Animals were not left behind, there were domestic animals roaming around the vicinity seeking for leftover to eat.

I saw our neighbour's hen, moving with her chicks towards the main road. She was trying to cross to the other side of the road which had a refuse dump. Suddenly, a fast-moving car hit her and three of her seven chicks. The Three chicks died on the spot, while others were unhurt. The hen also survived but with two smashed legs. I rush to the scene to confront the driver, but he zoomed off. I picked up the amputated hen, and some persons assisted me in catching the other four surviving chicks. And we took them home.

When the owner of the hen saw the magnitude of the injury, he ordered that the hen should be slaughtered immediately. It was clear that the hen would not survive the accident, even if she did, she would be useless. However, I pleaded that the hen should be taken care of, but he insisted that the hen should be used for pepper soup instantly. He was not even talking about the surviving chicks. I offered to buy the hen, and he concurred. The price was as if I was buying a dead hen, which I paid.

I had to chop off the pieces of the shattered legs to make it smooth. I kept applying traditional medicine on the hen's amputated legs, hoping it would get better. The chicks were too young to cope without their mother's care, so they all died few days after. Since she couldn't fend for herself due to her injuries, I had to feed her with crumbs of rice, bread and garri from our family rations. However, in a normal African family setting where poverty limits common men from having even two un-squared meals, I couldn't feed the hen consistently. How could I feed her, when my family sometimes did not have sufficient food for every member? Sometimes, the hen had to live for days without food. She kept struggling with hunger and pains, until the wound healed. She kept staying in the space that I kept her, waiting for my irregular suppliers.

My father went for a traditional marriage celebration and came back home with large chunks of rice that was served. Everyone at home ate to their satisfaction, and we still had leftover. The next morning, I happily rushed to see and feed my physically challenged hen, but I couldn't find her in the space she occupied. I hurriedly went to the open space at the front of our house to look for her. And behold, I saw her in the mist of other fowls; she was painstakingly scraping the ground with her blunt amputated knee in search of food. My knee became weak; tears filled my eyes, and I sat on a pavement and wept slowly.

The hen was tired of my inconsistent meals. She became fed up of her over dependence on someone. She has decided to run her life regardless of the pains ahead. She discovered that it is better to die trying than to live begging. The hen also understood that comfort zone is the burial ground of champions, while battlefields are the crucible where champions are made. She finally understood that there is no celebrated beggar anywhere, but celebrated givers. She also observed that the dependent can never be greater than his provider. And the receiver will always be the slave of the giver. I think she also knew that it is more honourable to eat an earned unbalanced food than to dine with the president without charge. Maybe, she later knew that over dependence leads to brain drain and destroys ingenuity.

The hen also discovered that the receiver cannot query the giver for what he gives. The giver will only give after he has satisfied his own wants. The giver cannot give his best; you will merely receive remainders. She noticed that it is better to face the challenges of fishing than to enjoy the partial sweetness of begged fishes. The hen understood that a dollar earned is far better than ten dollars found. She knew that the pains of starting would soon be overshadowed by the joy of success.

Few weeks after, the hen became pregnant and had ten chicks. She raised eight out of the ten to maturity without assistance from anyone.

Frustration/Joy

Helen Adams Keller

Deaf, Blind and Speech impediment

I was born on June 27, 1880, in Tuscumbia a little town of northern Alabama. My father Arthur was a captain in the confederate army and my mother who was much younger than him was his second wife. I was told that as an infant, I showed signs of eagerness to learn. I imitated anything I saw others do or say. They said at six months I could pipe out "How d, ye,"", meaning; How are you? And "Wah, wah", that is water. I was born with the ability to see and hear. I was completely healthy and sound indeed.

In February, 1882, I developed a severe congestion of the stomach and brain. Doctors called the sickness "brain fever", but did not give the cause of it. For several days, I suffered from high fever and severe pains in my eyes. Our family doctor thought I would die, but I didn't. The fever gradually subsided and I regained strength, nevertheless; my eyes continued to pain me. My eyes were so dry and hot that I had to turn to the wall to shade them from light. I woke up one day to discover that everywhere was dark and still. I went back to bed, assuming that it was still night. Morning never came, and I at no time hear the dinner bell again. That was how I started living in a world with neither light nor sound.

I noticed that people did not use signs as I did when they wanted anything done, but talk with their mouth. Sometimes I stood between people who were conversing touching their lips. I could not understand. I moved my lips frantically without result; this made me very angry and frustrated. I became quick-tempered and tormented my family members. I constantly smashed dishes, lamps and anything when angry. Some of my relatives called me monster and suggested that I should be taken to a mental institution. My mother felt helpless about how to deal with my destructive behaviour. She was always sad and sometimes wished for my death. The frustration at not being able to express myself intensified as I grew older. The darkness and dumbness of my world were boring and frustrating that sometimes I would scream and kick until I was exhausted. I nearly killed my kid sister, when I angrily overturned the cradle.

At age six, my family could no longer manage my frustration. My outburst increased from daily to hourly. My mother was afraid because I was capable of harming myself or anyone. With the assistance of Dr. Alexander Graham Bell, my family employed a teacher to teach me. The 20-year-old Anne Sullivan, herself visually impaired, became my instructor. The morning after my teacher came; she led me into her room and gave me a doll and she slowly spelt into my hands the word "d-o-l-l". I didn't know what she did, but she kept repeating it. She also tried other words like mug and water; all attempt failed. I couldn't comprehend what she was doing. I became impatient for her repeated attempts, and my intense frustration of not being able to communicate immediately crept in, seizing the new doll, I dashed it upon the floor.

My teacher knew that it would be impossible to teach a wild and tyrannical pupil like me. She then planned to win my love. Miss Annie did everything to make me happy, all to no avail. Her efforts suffered a major setback when she tried to discipline me for misbehaving; I assaulted her, knocking out one of her front teeth. In the mute, dark world in which I live, there was no strong sentiment or tenderness. My teacher spent a month with me, but I learnt nothing. My anger and frustration made me feel as if invisible hands were holding me, and I usually broke down in tears because I lacked the power to break free.

Miss Annie carefully discovered that I enjoyed going into the warm sunset. On a certain day, she gave me my hat, and I understood what she meant. The thought of taking a walk gave me a wordless feeling that made me hop and skip with pleasure. Joyfully we walked through the path to the well house. The fragrance of the honeysuckle and the fine, resinous odour of pine needles, blended with the perfumes of wild grapes gave me unspeakable happiness. Someone was drawing water, and my teacher placed my hand under the spout. As the cool streams gushed over one hand, she spelt into the other the word water, first slowly, then rapidly. I stood still; my whole attention focused upon the motions of her finger. Suddenly, I felt a misty consciousness of something forgotten, a thrill of returning thoughts and somehow the mystery of language was revealed to me. I knew then that water was the name of the wonderful cool thing that was flowing over my hand. That living word awakened my soul, gave it light, hope, and joy and set it free.

I left the well house eager to learn because I knew now that everything has a name. As we return to the house every object which I touched seems to quiver with life. This was because I saw everything with the strange fresh sight that has come to me. I learnt a great many new words that day. I know that father, mother, sister, teacher were among them. From that day, my soul was awakened, I did nothing but explore with my hands and learnt the name of every object that I touched; and the more I handed things and know their names and uses; the more joyous and confident grew my sense of relationship with the rest of the world. As my knowledge of things grew, I learnt more and more words; gradually, my field of inquiry broadened. I soon learnt how to read. My teacher gave me slips of cardboard on which were printed words in raised letters. Thus, I began to read.

With a burning desire to learn more, I desperately yearned to attend a conventional school. Therefore, in 1888 and 1894, I attended the Perkins Institute for the Blind and Wright-Humason School for the Deaf. In 1896, I entered The Cambridge School for Young Ladies before gaining admittance, in 1900, to Radcliffe College. In 1904, at the age of 24, I graduated from Radcliffe, becoming the first deaf-blind person to earn a Bachelor of Arts degree.

Before her death in 1968, Miss Keller received honorary doctoral degrees from Temple and Harvard Universities in the United States; Glasgow and Berlin Universities in Europe; Delhi University in India; and Witwatersrand University in South Africa. She won numerous honours, including Lions Humanitarian Award, the Presidential Medal of Freedom, and election to the Women's Hall of Fame. Her birthday on June 27 is commemorated as Helen Keller Day in the U.S. state of Pennsylvania. She *wrote* eight *books* that got translated into over 50 languages. In her lifetime, she met all the presidents of the United States of America since Grover Cleveland.

Lesson 5

We live in our minds than in our bodies. The quality of our minds determines the worth of our life. But the condition of our body can never determine the worth of our life. The state of our mind always affects our physical appearance, but our physique has little or no effect on our minds. Majority of man's invention started from the mind before it was produced with the hands. Sound mind leads to good life, but a completely active body can never guarantee a pleasant life. It is better to have a sound mind than a good physique. Someone else can assist you in carrying out your physical responsibility, but no one can reason for you. Therefore, it is important to protect your mind.

Anger will never change the circumstances, rather it would hurt you, and the challenge would remain. The angrier you are the more disable you become. A man who cannot control his physical and mental state is totally out of action. Already you are physically challenged; anger and frustration are mental disabilities, thereby making you completely incapacitated. Physical disability can be very frustrating, but when combined with mental disability, life becomes tasteless. Productivity is of the mind than it is of the body. The reason why we are not productive is that we allow our physical challenges to determine the state of our mind. A furious man would never think well.

Your parents may have been the cause of your challenge, because they failed to give you proper medication. Your company might have been the reason, because you were exposed to diverse workplace hazards. A reckless driver may perhaps be the rationale for your problems. Fighting for your country might be the agent of your unfavourable condition. Maybe, you are blaming your creator. The truth is; the earlier you stop blaming the cause of your challenge the better your life would be. Blaming and regret is one of the root causes of anger. Your physical state might be terrible, but if you can keep your mind in good shape, your life will not be like your physique.

Anger puts off the brain. That is why people regret their anger triggered actions afterwards, because they were not thinking when the deeds were done. An anxious man can never be productive. Learning will be very difficult for a turbulent mind. An angry mind can never produce anything good; its products are hatred, sorrow, regret, discontent, hopelessness and even suicide. All inventions of the world came from calm minds. Creative thinkers prefer to work or live in quit environments, to enable them effectively arrange their thoughts. However, the greatest noise doesn't come from the environment; it comes from within. A graveyard can be as noisy as Wall Street for a troubled mind.

The world you once greatly enjoyed has suddenly become unfavourable, just be calm. The people you were assisting are now insulting you; be quiet. Your once lovely physique has been shattered, relax. Your finance is not as huge as it used to be, don't worry. You can't do what others do, calm down. You have suddenly become an object of mockery, be still. A planet full of anger will never solve a handful of problem.

Self Pity

Stephen Hawking

Paralysis

For an extra ordinary research work on Cosmology, I received my PhD from Cambridge in 1962 at age 23. Since then, I have received increasing global academic recognition of my work in Physics and Cosmology that has resulted to awards and honours. In 1979, two years after I was appointed a professor in gravitational physics, I received the Albert Einstein Medal and an honorary doctorate from the University of Oxford. In 1982 The British Government honoured me with The Order of the British Empire (Commander). And in 2009, I won the Presidential Medal of Freedom, the highest civilian honour in the United States by President

Barack Obama.

Other awards include; Eddington Medal (1975), Hughes Medal of the Royal Society (1976) , Franklin Medal(1981),Gold Medal of the Royal Astronomical Society(1985), Member of the Pontifical Academy of Sciences (1986), Wolf Prize in Physics(1988), Prince of Asturias Awards in Concord(1989), Companion of Honour(1989) , Julius Edgar Lilienfeld Prize of the American Physical Society(1999) ,Michelson Morley Award of Case Western Reserve University(2003),Copley Medal of the Royal Society(2006), Fonseca Price of the University of Santiago de Compostela (2008).

I have also written few books, one of them "A brief history of life" which has already been translated into 33 languages and has sold more than nine million copies. Due to my wide range of research work and imaginative power, people say I am an equal to only Sir Isaac Newton and Albert Einstein. All these awards and achievement would have been a mirage if not for a sight in 1963 at St Bartholomew's Hospital.

I was born on the 8th of January in the year 1942 in Oxford, England. Although, I did not have a strong body from childhood; I was weak and had some problems with my speech, but I was a normal child. My father introduced me to survey and astronomy at a very tender age. My family loves education; therefore, we spent most of our time at home reading. I had a close group of friends with whom I enjoyed board games. I and my friend; John built model seaplanes and airplanes. Although at school, I was known as "Einstein," I was initially not successful academically. With time, I began to show considerable aptitude for scientific subjects, and I decided to study mathematics at university.

I arrived at the University College in 1959, at age 17, several years younger than most of my fellow students. The curriculum of my course of study was okay and easy going. The duration of my course of study at Cambridge was three years and in my final year, I had started making plans for my graduate studies. In this last year of studies, I noticed that I seem to be getting clumsier, and I fell over once or twice for no apparent reason. I also discovered I had difficulty rowing a sculling boat. For some reasons, I decided to hide these symptoms from my family and some of my friends. One day, I fell down a flight of stairs, landing on my head. It took me several hours to recover all my memory. At a point, my health deteriorated that I couldn't hide it from my family members anymore. I was totally losing balance. My mother was so worried that she insisted that I see the family doctor.

Shortly after my 21st birthday, I entered St Bartholomew's Hospital. I spent two weeks undergoing series of unpleasant medical tests. They took a muscle sample from my arm, stuck electrodes into me, and injected some radio-opaque fluid into my spine, and watched it going up and down with x-rays, as they slanted the bed. After all the tests, the doctors shocked me by informing me that I had contracted 'Amyotrophic lateral sclerosis (A.L.S). 'A.L.S' is a type of neuromuscular disease that gradually weakens muscular strength and the nerves of the spinal cord. As a result of A.L.S, body cells lose their strength over time and cause muscle paralysis, and the brain loses its control over the body muscles. They say that the disease was almost incurable and there was nothing they could do for me except to give me vitamins. I gathered that the disease would continue to get worse; literally, it was a kind of slow death. And the doctors predicted two more years for me to live.

Upon hearing the doctor's heart-rending report I became terribly traumatized and depressed. "How could something like this happen to me?" was my question. I had no reason to continue my graduate programme when I would not live to complete it. In truth, there was no reason to live. I started having series of nightmares; one of them was dreaming that I was going to be executed. Indulging in activities that could help me forget the painful feelings of my forthcoming death was fruitless. I even thought of sacrificing my life to save others because I was going to die. I felt sorry for my unfortunate life and got bored with life. I withdrew from my friends and family.

However, while I was in the hospital, I saw a boy I vaguely knew dying of leukaemia in the bed opposite me, and it was not a good-looking sight. This singular view transformed my life. Life immediately came back to me. Clearly, there were people who were worse off than me. I instantly went back to Cambridge and carried on with the research I had just started in general relativity and cosmology. Although the diseases made it difficult for me to walk and to hold things properly, but I always remember that I am better than some persons. Instead of pitying myself, I laboriously continued and finished the research work on

Cosmology.

Although, today I can no longer speak, move or drive my wheelchair independently, but I am enjoying a rich, fulfilling life, because I know I'm better than so many people. The doctors said I would not see my twenty third birthday, but today I am more than fifty years old. I have had a full and satisfying life.

Lesson 6

If you want to beg or depend on others to survive forever, keep pitying yourself. Self sympathy is the bedrock of begging among the physically challenged. You seek assistance from people because you feel they are better than you. When you keep blaming your physical challenge for your economic or social woos, you are afflicted with "self pity syndrome." Like a virus, it spreads to all the parts of your body, and it becomes incurable when it gets to the brain. That is why we have professional beggars who have dumped diverse opportunities to become self-reliant for begging.

This feeling does not only consume the person interiorly but seems to make him a burden to others. The person feels condemned to receive help and assistance from others and at the same time seems useless to himself.

Self-pity kills ingenuity. Instead of channelling your time and strength to productive thinking, self-pity makes you spend time on complains, regret and wishes. Feeling inferior can lead to depression and depression is the highway to sickness and death. It makes you feel worthless. Don't let anyone pity you because humans are not constant. People can be compassionate today and unfeeling tomorrow. They might be sympathetic for some time but change later. Your relatives or friends might pay your bills for few years; believe me, they will get tired someday. If you let them pity you, they will weaken your ability to cater for yourself.

You are not meant to be pitied but to be envied. There are people you are far better than. Some physically challenged are praying to be like you. If you are blind, somebody is blind-deaf. If you lost two arms, someone doesn't have arms and legs. If you are paralysed someone is living on life support. If you are on life support, remember that someone in that same hospital died today. You have every reason to be glad.

Advantage

Thomas Alva Edison

Deaf

Thomas Edison's childhood was a bittersweet experience. His father Sam Edison was a prosperous lumber and feed dealer in Milan, Ohio. The Edison's fortunes declined due to the reduction of canal tariffs at Milan in competition with the railroad and depression in the town.

The family moved to Port Huron, which had a positive economic potential. At the age of eleven Thomas decided to venture into business to enable him to raise money to support his family and meet his laboratory needs. Edison sold vegetables like onions, lettuce, cabbages and peas around town. Later, he sold candy, fruits, butter, newspapers and magazines on trains running from Port Huron to Detroit.

Although Thomas' official schooling lasted for just three months, learning was the game he loved. Edison kept reading books on literature and science. Edison was able to make himself a laboratory in the back of the train where he conducted experiments. He also had plans to go back to school after his family's finance stabilizes.

Then, as if to make life harder for Tom, there came the cruel affliction of deafness. His deafness seems to have been traceable to the after effect of scarlet fever Thomas suffered immediately his family arrived at Port Huron. He was thus permanently disabled at age 13. It became virtually impossible for him to acquire knowledge in a typical educational setting for he would not hear his teachers. The prospect of a handicapped lad of a poor family was certainly not good.

Amazingly, he never seemed to fret a whole lot over the matter. He saw and focused on the advantage of the loss of his hearing. Now he could concentrate, could think something through without interruption. This calamity drove him to more sustained efforts at reading, reflecting and studying. He began to learn absolutely everything by himself. There were fewer distractions, so Tom spent and enjoyed so many hours alone, wholly lost in his elementary experiments with wet cells and stovepipe wire and his first crude telegraph instruments.

Thomas paid the two-dollar fee and became a patron of the Detroit Public Library. Given that he couldn't hear what people say, he spent his spare time studying rather than conversing with friends. Tom started with the first book on the bottom shelf and went through the group, one by one. He didn't read a few books; he read the library. With aggressive crave for knowledge, Thomas devoured books on electricity, mechanics, chemical analysis, manufacturing, technology and more. Thus, the loss of his hearing brought him, to an important positive turning point in his life.

At age 15, he discovered that deafness was an advantage to a telegrapher. While he could hear unerring the loud ticking of the instrument, he could not hear other and perhaps distracting sounds. Thomas decided to become a telegrapher. At the age of 19, Tom has become a genius in telegraphy, it was said, and he had few equals. Thanks to ceaseless self-education and mechanically experiment. It was during these years of self-education that he acquired experience that made him an inventor. And at age 23, Thomas Edison designed his first operative invention; the electric vote recorder. Shortly thereafter, he was absolutely astonished, in fact; he nearly fainted when a corporation paid him $40,000 for all of his rights to his new invention; the Stock-Ticker.

The world of Science, business and invention would be incomplete without mentioning the name; Thomas Edison. Before he died in 1931, Edison patented 1,093 of his inventions. The wonders of his mind include the microphone, telephone receiver, universal stock ticker, phonograph, kinetoscope, storage battery, electric pen, and mimeograph. Regardless of his deafness, Edison established himself as one of the most prolific inventors of all time.

Lesson 7

The society sometimes feels that the physically challenge has nothing good to offer. Therefore, when any physically challenged person disapproves this belief, he becomes a celebrity instantly. Most world celebrities wouldn't have been famous if they were not physically challenged. People celebrate folks that overcame diverse challenges to gain success.

Focusing on the disability of a part of the body, leads to disability of the whole body. Instead focus on your areas of ability and the advantages of your disability. Stop complaining about what you cannot do, become perfect in what you can do. Everything that has disadvantages also has advantages. Concentrating on the negative effect of an occurrence instead of the positive aspect is the reason why people are incapacitated.

When you start with disadvantage, you have to work harder to do what others take for granted. In the end that gives you an advantage. You have learnt to go the extra mile to stretch yourself further than you envisioned was possible. Your meticulousness will make you better than others. Instead of discouraging you, let your physical challenge motivate you to work harder than others.

It would be thoughtless to assume that disability is better than wholeness. It would also be ignorance to guess that any part of the body is irrelevant. However, we cannot as well overlook the peaceful and quiet world of the deaf, which gives room for concentration and rational thinking. The dark world of the blind is the birth place of innovative imagination that can touch the world positively. If you can think well, you will see at least one benefit of your condition. Ensure you effectively utilize the advantages of your challenges and pay less attention to your disabilities.

Endurance/Persistence

Pope John Paul 11

Parkinson's disease

The world came to a halt on 13 May, 1981, the day sixty years-old Pope John Paul 11 was shot and critically wounded by Mehmet Ali as he entered St. Peter's Square to address an audience. On the way to Gemelli Hospital, he lost consciousness because he had lost almost three-quarters of his blood, near exsanguinations.

At that moment, the world was divided into two: one part praying that the Pope should live, while the other wished him dead. The Communist government in Central and Eastern Europe, especially in Poland knew he was their key threat. While the oppressed people of Central and Eastern Europe knew he was their major support and inspiration in their quest to reinstall democracy, freedom and human rights. His open criticism of apartheid South Africa made him an enemy of the white majority, whereas he remained a source of strength for Nelson Mandela, Desmond Tutu and the blacks in South Africa. Mafia groups in Southern Italy recognised that his active fights against them will lead to their fall, while victims of mafia violence wanted him to intensify his efforts. Even the Papacy had two factions; those that disliked his constant appointment of Africans, Americans and North Europeans to high Vatican posts and others that appreciated his non-discrimination against races.

Pope John Paul 11 was born Karol Józef Wojtyła on 18 May 1920 in the Polish town of Wadowice. He attended Jagiellonian University where he studied philology and various languages. After Nazi German occupation forces closed the university after invading Poland and the sudden death of his father, he decided to become a priest. On finishing his studies at the seminary in Kraków, Wojtyła was ordained as a priest on All Saints' Day, 1 November 1946, by the Archbishop of Kraków, Cardinal Sapieha. John Paul became the bishop of Ombi in 1958 and then the archbishop of Krakow six years later. In 1978, John Paul made history by becoming the first non-Italian pope in more than four hundred years and the first from Poland.

Since his pontificate, he has dedicated his life to charity. His compassion for the oppressed, poor, sick, elderly, discriminated and afflicted made him visit many countries to spread the message of hope and peace. He shunned the trappings that came with his position as Pope. His sympathy for the sick, the old and physically challenged made him visit countless hospitals and homes to give comfort and support to the physically and mentally challenged. He also visited various prisons, advocating for better prison conditions, fair trial and abolishment of capital punishment. A strong advocate for human rights, he visited more than

100 countries speaking against corruption, discrimination and war.

He became the hope to the oppressed, sick, prisoners and discriminated. Pope John Paul was an agent of change, every country he visited experienced positive changes. Christians and people of other religions prayed for the Pope to visit their country because he was courageous enough to criticise any inhuman government.

His Holiness miraculously survived the attack. He underwent five hours of surgery to treat his wounds and spent 22 days in the hospital being treated for abdominal wounds and blood infection. He recovered fully, but his health never remained the same. Pope John Paul has been physically injured severely, and his health gradually declined. Pope John Paul was later diagnosed of Parkinson's disease; a nervous disease which spreads slowly through the body, causing trembling of limbs and head. Symptoms can be partially controlled by drugs, but there is no known cure. The Pope started showing signs of Parkinson's, including slurred speech and trembling. And he could no longer walk and sometimes had difficulty speaking and hearing.

However, it was evident that in his pains and sufferings, the Pope was resolute in working the hardest he could to keep spreading the message of peace and love. Instead of taking things slow for a while, he maintained his zeal. When one is under pain and has difficulty doing what once came so easily, temptation to give up will arouse, but the pope courageously continued to do what he loved. He endured the pains and suffering of sickness just to ensure that he put smiles in the faces of the downtrodden.

In poor health John Paul the Great gave hope and strength to the sick and the elderly. He visited countless hospitals and homes in various continents giving people reasons to live. His physicians kept advising him to reduce his journey, but all were futile. He once said that "It is wonderful to be able to give oneself to the very end for the sake of the kingdom of God" Despite difficulty speaking more than a few sentences at a time, trouble hearing and severe osteoarthrosis, he continued to tour the world, although rarely walking in public. Even when the sickness became unbearable, His Holiness refused to resign because he knew there was still much work to be done. He was one of the most travelled world leaders in history, visiting 129 countries during his pontificate.

His achievements in the period of good health cannot be compared to his giant strides in his days of affliction. He was active in service until he neared death.

Against all odds, the Pope appeared at his apartment window March 30 2005; His Holiness greeted pilgrims in St. Peter's Square and tried in vain to speak to them. After four minutes, he was wheeled from view, and the curtains of his apartment window were drawn. And the next day following a urinary tract infection, he developed septic shock, a form of infection with a high fever and low blood pressure. The pope died on April 2, 2005 at 9:37 p.m. But the day before his death, he was able to concelebrate Mass in his papal apartment.

His burial in 2005 was the single largest gathering of heads of state in history. Four kings, five queens, at least 70 presidents and prime ministers, and more than 14 leaders of other religions attended. It is likely to have been the largest single pilgrimage of Christianity ever, with numbers estimated in excess of four million mourners gathering in Rome. His fame is not a product of his title as the head of the Catholic Church but the creation of his persistence to eradicate sorrow and oppression in spite of his own pains and sufferings.

Lesson 8

For the newborn to travel from the womb to the point of delivery, he must endure hardship and pains. The mother also must persistently 'push' regardless of the unbearable pains of labour. The seed must persistently push the earth crust to enable its seedling to see the sun. The gasp for breath, the jerk of the body, the squeezing of certain body parts and the gradual disappearance of the eye pupil shows that death is also painful. Suffering is part of human existence from birth until death, and every human person suffers in a variety of ways: physically, psychologically, socially, and spiritually. No matter how terrible you think your pain is, someone has undergone or is undergoing greater pains.

If we keep considering the pains of suffering, life will be meaningless because we will achieve nothing. The fear of the pains of child birth will make a woman barren. The horror of circumcision would not stop a parent from circumcising their male child. The pains of the body must not stop us from pursuing our goals and purpose. We can endure the pains. There is no unbearable pain.

The author Victor Frankel in his book Man's Search for Meaning describes his horrifying experiences in Nazi concentration camps. He notes that although all the prisoners were in the same material circumstances like; danger of death, the death of relatives or friends, amputation of body organs, disease, sexual abuse, homesickness, persecution, mockery, scorn, loneliness, abandonment and the most horrible imaginable condition. Yet, they did not all react in the same way. Some prisoners killed themselves by walking into electrified fences; others clung to life and even found joy despite the atrocities occurring around them daily. What made the difference? One way to put it is that man can endure anything if he has a reason to live. Conversely, man can endure nothing if he does not.

Some physical challenged people kill themselves; others become addicts, and many prefer depression because they have nothing to live for. Others decide to suffer the pains and persistently pursue their purpose. The state of disability is not your destination, but a bus stop you must laboriously run the race persistently to reach your end in order to wear your crown of fame. Life is not a bed of roses but with endurance and persistence, you can make it rosy.

Love/Giving

Nick Vujicic

Limbless

My parents were very expectant that important morning of 13th March 1982 when my mother was rushed to the hospital due to labour pains. My father, who was present when I was born, was so shocked when he saw me that he had to leave the hospital room to vomit. My distressed mother couldn't bring herself to hold me. I was like a monster; nobody in my family has ever seen a human without arms and legs. I had no limb except a small foot on my left hip that has two toes. There was no medical explanation for my condition; doctors only said it was a rare occurrence called Phocomelia. It took so much courage for my mother to hold me when I was four months.

Instead of celebrating my birth, my Parents, relatives and friends mourned. My parents spent many years asking why this unkind thing would happen to them. When they knew that they cannot change anything, they accepted me wholeheartedly. They began to devise various styles and devices that would make me live an independent life. My dad put me in the water at 18 months and gave the courage to learn to swim. My mother invented a special plastic device that assisted me in holding pen with my two toes.

As a boy, I spent many nights praying for limbs. I will go to sleep crying and dream that I would wake up to find they had miraculously appeared. It never happened. As I grew up, I became convinced that there was nothing good about me; I felt I was totally useless. My inability to see a future ahead coupled with ceaseless bullying at school made me extremely depressed. In school, I was treated like an alien; my classmates kept their distance.

When I was ten years old, I decided to end my life by drowning myself in a bathtub, but I couldn't. The truth was that I disliked myself. As I moved into my teen years, I gradually won acceptance, first from myself and then others. I decided to be thankful for what I do have, not get angry about what I don't. 'I looked at myself in the mirror and said: 'you know what; the world is right that I have no arms or legs, but they'll never take away the beauty of my eyes.' I also realised that I have blessing, talent, knowledge and love to share with others. These truths made me fall in love with myself. From this time, I never focused on my abbreviated body anymore. I summoned courage to strike conversations with people. The more I did this, the more they accepted that I was not an alien dropped into their mist.

Apart from prayer, the action that gave my life meaning is giving. I discovered that the more I dwelt on my challenges, the worse I felt, but when I changed my focus to serving the needs of someone else, it lifted my spirits and help me understand that no one suffers alone. My parents were not rich, so I could not give financial assistance to the needy, but I have something to offer, which is inspiring those in need. Regardless of my physical challenge, I could write, type, and swim. I had also learnt to do a lot of the daily things a normal person can do, like answer the phone, shave, brush my teeth, comb my hair and get a glass of water. Instead of discussing my problems and challenges with people I decided to inspire them by telling them how I overcome adversities. Instead of attracting pity, I decided to be a blessing.

In time, these discussions with classmates on overcoming adversities led to invitations for me to speak to students groups, church youth groups and other teen organisations. People were willing to listen to me because they know I faced and overcome my challenges. Instinctively, people felt I might have something to say that could help them with their own problems. In one of such meetings within the first three minutes of my talk, half the girls were crying, and most of the boys were struggling to hold their emotions together. One girl, in particular, was sobbing very hard. We all looked at her, and she put her hand up. She said, "I am so sorry to interrupt, but can I come up and hug you?" She came hugged me in front of everyone, and whispered in my ear, "Thank you, thank you, thank you. No one has ever told me that they loved me, and that I am beautiful the way I am."

While majoring in both accountancy and financial planning at a university, I also worked on developing my abilities as a speaker. My desire to give has inspired me to go across 44 countries and sharing the message of hope to over 5 million people. Today my Life without Limbs non-profit organisation helps support more than ten different charities around the world. I am happy, independent and married with a son.

Lesson 9

You cannot be loved more than you love yourself. Nobody would honour you greater than the level you grant yourself. You are the best marketer of yourself. What you showcase is what people accept. You would never receive from others what you have not given to yourself. If you dislike the way you look, people would follow suit. If you feel you are inferior, the world would feel the same. If you show people that you are useless because you are physically challenged, they would treat you like one.

Stop wishing to be someone else or to reverse your past. Don't pretend to be who you are not. Most people hide their disability because they are ashamed of themselves. You are unique and still relevant; nobody can do what you can do. There can never be another you.

Love yourself, give yourself, honour yourself, accept yourself, respect yourself and others will.

After you have accepted yourself, help others gain control of their lives. You will never suffer what we give. In your challenge give hope to others. Encourage people that are going through what you are undergoing. In your financial struggle give little to people in need. Instead of feeding people with pathetic stories of your problems, tell them heroic stories of how you were able to overcome your challenges. Instead of attracting sympathy, draw inspiration. Share any little accomplishment with people. Tell them how you were able to accomplish a task without assistance. As you passionately do this, your suffering would gradually fade away.

One of the ways of distinguishing yourself from the dependent nature of the physically challenge is to give. As a substitute of being always the receiver, become the giver. Dedicate your effort and time thinking and devising ways to put smiles on people's face. Regardless of your pains, focus on developing products and services that would make the world a better place. As you keep giving, you would gradually have reasons for living. As you constantly give, your deliverance from the beggarly life of most physically challenged persons would be accomplished.

Start Again

Earvin "Magic" Johnson

HIV

"**I** do have concerns, just like anybody would have. Look at the cuts and scratches I get now, It is a physical game, and you do get kicked and scratched, I have concerns about the possibility of being infected while playing with Magic", this was the comment of Karl Malone, who plays for the Utah Jazz. Several NBA players had also said recently that they were concerned about playing against Johnson for fear of contracting the virus. One NBA general manager, speaking on the condition, told the New York Times that Johnson should step aside to avoid any controversy.

Despite reassurance by many notable physicians

like William Reiter, the Director of Clinical Research at the Center for Special Immunology that they have nothing to fear by playing against Magic, many players stated that they would be hesitant to guard him. During a preseason game Magic Johnson injured himself and many players refused to continue the game on account of the blood from Johnson's injury possibly infecting another player. When Magic announced that he would participate in the Olympics, Immediately Australian players protested, saying they would not play against Magic.

This was the challenge of Earvin Johnson, a three-time NBA "Most Valuable Player" and 12-time All-Star team member. His passing, dribbling skills, and ballhandling technique won him the nickname "Magic." His magnetic personality made him one of the most popular players in the league. Referred as one of the greatest basketball players of all time, Johnson spent his entire 13-season NBA career with the Lakers, helping them to win five championships in the 1980s.

Johnson's joy turned to sorrow before the 1991–92 NBA season, when he discovered that he had tested positive for HIV. He also understood that it is simply impossible to play in the NBA without creating controversies and there was nothing he could do about it. Magic was forced to resign at the prime of his career. It was a sad retirement. During his playing career, Magic earned just over $18 million in salary and several million more in endorsements. He was out of job and has a family to support.

Many sports analysts and fans wondered what Johnson would do as he had retired from basketball with just over $ 18 million. Some expected that he would soon file for bankruptcy like other stars that their careers were short-lived.

He sat down and thought of what else he could venture in to sustain himself and family. Johnson discovered that he could do business. Therefore, he decided to start a new life in the business world. Johnson curtailed the flamboyant life style lived by NBA stars to prove his readiness to be a businessman. His new personality began to attract businesses to him. In 1990 he purchased the Pepsi-Cola distribution plant in Forestville, Maryland, with the assistance of Black Enterprise publisher, Earl G. Graves. He channelled his NBA magic style to business and within few years, Johnson began to make profitable marks in business.

Today Magic Johnson Enterprises is valued at over $1 billion and has given Johnson a personal net worth of $500 million, making him the second richest NBA star of all times after Michael Jordan. He occupies the fifth position in Forbes's ranking of the 20 wealthiest black Americans. Magic Johnson Enterprises owns Magic Johnson Theatres, a nationwide chain of movie theatres; and Magic Johnson Entertainment, a film studio. In 1994, Magic paid $10 million to buy 4.5% of The Lakers which he sold in 2010 to billionaire Patrick Soon-Shiong for a reported $50-60 million. In 2010, Johnson also sold his chain of Starbucks for $75 million.

He also invested in urban real estate and a company catering to America's underserved markets via his Canyon-Johnson and Yucaipa-Johnson funds. On March 27, 2012, Magic and a group of partners purchased The Los Angeles Dodgers from Frank McCourt for $2 Billion. Johnson created the Magic Johnson Foundation to help combat HIV and undertake other charitable endeavours, and he has awarded more than $1.1 million to community-based organizations that focus on HIV/AIDS education and prevention. His determination to start over again has made him richer than many NBA stars that retired at old age.

Lesson 10

Discrimination against people with disability might never end. It will take decades or even centuries to greatly reduce disability prejudice. Regardless of world's effort to eradicate racial and gender discrimination, they still persist. One of the cardinal triggers of discrimination is fear. People do not really dislike the physically challenged; they are just scared of their capacity. People feel that because a part of one's body is disabled, then everything about him is out of action. Employers are afraid to employ the physically challenged not because they are unqualified, but because they doubt their abilities. Only few passengers will comfortably board a bus or plane if they were informed that the driver or pilot is physically challenged.

We don't necessarily need to aggressively collide with our challenges to overcome them. Sometimes we don't even need to fight discrimination openly to win it. We can defeat discrimination by withdrawing to reinforce. Retreating to strengthen is not cowardice but moving back permanently is. When you don't currently have enough strength or power to overcome existing discrimination; withdraw, reinforce and re-attack. Reinforce by improving your education, embarking on relevant training, acquiring more skills, self-employment, innovation, and new discoveries. It might take time, but victory will be sure. Remember attacking a well-armed enemy unarmed might be disastrous.

When your physical challenge makes it difficult for you to continue your job, search for an alternative. You can also invent an advanced way of performing the job. However, instead of wasting time pleading to be retained or employed, there are some other tasks you can do. We have multiple talents but a definite purpose. Each of our talent is a pathway to our purpose.

Therefore, if it is impossible to develop a particular talent because of your physical challenge, you have to discover and develop other talents you possess. Don't waste so much time wishing that the organisation's policies will be changed to suit your condition. If the organisation decides to disengage you, life must move on. Engage yourself in other productive activities. Like Magic Johnson, you might buy up or become the owner of the firm that once threw you out.

Bibliography

Ajayi, O. (2012, February 17). *Interview: Nigeriafilms.com* . Retrieved from NFC Media Group: www.nigeriafilms.com

Anderson, P. M. (1995). Cautious Defense: Should I be Afraid to Guard You? (Mandatory AIDS Testing in Proffessional Team Sports). *Marquette University Sport Law Review*, 279-314.

Attitude is Altitude Organisation. (2013). *About Nick: Attitude is Altitude Organisation*. Retrieved from Attitude is Altitude Web site: www.attitudeisaltitude.com

Beals, G. (1999, June). *The Biography of Thomas Edison: Brocktonma Corporation.* Retrieved from Brocktonma Corporation Web site: www.brocktonma.com

British Broadcasting Corporation. (2001, January 3). *BBC News/Europe/Pope has Parkinson's disease-surgeon.* Retrieved from BBC Web site: bbc.co.uk

Cable News Network. (2011, December 20th). *edition.cnn.com/africanvoice.* Retrieved from Turner Broadcasting System, Inc.: www.cnn.com

Catholic News Service/U.S. Conference of Catholic Bishops. (2005). *Pope John Paul II's Final Days:American Catholic Organisation.* Retrieved from American Catholic Organisation Web site: www.americancatholic.org

Celebrity Net Worth. (2013, December 20). *Magic Johnson Net Worth:Celebrity Net Worth.* Retrieved from Celebrity Net Worth Web site: http//www.Celebritynetworth.com

Chicago Tribune. (2008, June 29). *News: Chicago Tribune.* Retrieved from Chicago Tribune Website: chicagotribune.com

Cobhams Asuquo Music Productions. (2008). *News: Cobhams Asuquo Music Productions.* Retrieved from Cobhams Asuquo Music Productions Web site: camp.com.ng

Forbes. (2009, June 5). *The Wealthiest Black Americans: Forbes.* Retrieved from Forbes Web site: http//www.forbes.com

Franklin D. Roosevelt Presidential Library and Museum. (2013, October 24). *About fdr/biographiesandmore: Franklin D. Roosevelt Presidential Library and Museum.* Retrieved from Franklin D. Roosevelt Presidential Library and Museum Web site: http://www.fdrlibrary.marist.edu

Franklin D. Roosevelt American Heritage Center, Inc. (2007). *About FDR: Franklin D. Roosevelt American Heritage Center, Inc.* Retrieved from Franklin D. Roosevelt American Heritage Center, Inc.: fdrheritage.org

Gibson, W. (Director). (1962). *The Miracle Worker* [Motion Picture].

Hawking, S. (2013). *My Brief History.* Bantam.

Herrmann, D., Keller, H., & Shattuck, R. (1903). *The Story of my Life.* New York: Doubleday, Page & CO.

Josephson, M. (1959). *A Select Edition of Edison: A Biography.* United States of America: McGraw-Hill Book Company and Harold Ober Associate, Inc.

Kaczor, C. (2013). A Pope's Answer to the Problem of Pain. *Catholic Answers Magazine*, p. Volume 18 Number 1.

Leprosy-Wikipedia, the free encyclopedia. (2013, October 1st). Retrieved from Wikipedia Corporation Web site: www.wikipedia.org

Mail Foreign Service. (2009 , July 1). *News: Associated Newspapers Ltd.* Retrieved from Associated Newspapers Ltd Web site: www.and.co.uk

Naaman-Wikipedia, the free encyclopedia. (2013, October 1st). Retrieved from Wikipedia Corporation Web site: www.wikipedia.com

Olatunji, S. (2011, September 11). *entertainment: Nigeriabestforum.* Retrieved from Nigerian Best Forum Website: www.nigerianbestforum.com

Palmer, R. (2013, September 17). *Tech / SciScience/Stephen Hawking Memoir My Brief History.* Retrieved from IBT Media Inc. Web site: ibtimes.com

The Holy Bible : Authorized King James Version. (2006). Nashville, Tennessee, United States of America: Holman Bible Publishers.

Thomson, C. (2013). *Mordecai Brown:sabr.org.* Retrieved from Society for American Baseball Research Web site: sabr.org

Vujicic, N. (2010). *Life Without Limits.* New York: Doubleday Religion.

Weiss, T. C. (2011, June 23). *Editorials/ Disabled World.* Retrieved from Disabled World Web site: www.disabled-world.com

Wikimedia Foundation Inc. (2013, November 27). *Pope John Paul II: Wikipedia, the free encyclopedia.* Retrieved from Wikipedia Web site: www.wikipedia.org

Wikipedia Corporation. (2013, November 9). *Franklin D. Roosevelt: Wikipedia, the free encyclopedia.* Retrieved from Wikipedia Corporation Web Site: www.wikipedia.org

Wikipedia Corporation. (2013, November 14). *Helen Keller: Wikipedia, the free encyclopedia.* Retrieved from Wikipedia Web site: www.wikipedia.org

Zenit News Agency. (2008, October 17). *Articles/film-reveals-john-paul-ii-s-courage-says-pope: Zenit News Agency* . Retrieved from Zenit News Agency Web site: http://www.zenit.org